THE VEGAN LIFESTYLE

Health Benefits of Being Vegan And Why is More Than A Diet with Delicious Plant-Based Recipes To Lose Weight And Satisfy Craving

By

Andrew Low

Table of Contents

Introduction

More people across the world discover the importance of vegan lifestyle and whole food plant-based diet when you eat healthy vegan foods, you are getting much more benefits that you can ever imagine:

1. Prevent Or Even Reverse Deadly Diseases:

   According to many studies, animal fats and meats might actually cause so many diseases such as diabetes, cancer, hypertension, heart diseases... Not to mention that some U.S studies showed that people who eat processed meats die prematurely and more frequently than other people.

2. Lose Fat And Get Fit:

   With the vegan diet, you can say goodbye to calorie restriction, body shaming or eating disorders. Plants contain fewer calories and more fiber and antioxidants than the animal -based products.

3. Improve and Protect the Environment:

One of the best benefits that the vegan diet offers is improving the Environment that ensures us and our children a better life because the production of meat and products that includes it requires lot of work and time that often caused so many people on the planet to starve because all their crops are sold to feed animals in other places to produce more meat and milk whereas they can live a simple life in peace and harmony by embracing the plant based diet.

SUMMARY OF HEALTH BENEFITS

Plant-based nutrition has exploded in popularity, and many advantages have been well documented over the past several decades. Not only is there a broad expansion of the research database supporting the myriad benefits of plant-based diets, but also health care practitioners are seeing awe-inspiring results with their patients across multiple unique subspecialties. Plant-based diets have been associated with lowering overall and ischemic heart disease mortality; supporting sustainable weight management; reducing medication needs; lowering the risk for most chronic diseases; decreasing the incidence and severity of high-risk conditions, including obesity, hypertension, hyperlipidemia, and hyperglycemia; and even possibly reversing advanced coronary artery disease and type 2 diabetes. The reason for these outcomes is twofold. First, there are inherent benefits to eating a wide variety of health-promoting plants. Second, there is additional benefit from crowding out—and thereby avoiding—the injurious constituents found in animal products, including the following:

- Saturated fats: Saturated fats are a group of fatty acids found primarily in animal products (but also in the plant kingdom—mostly in tropical oils, such as coconut and palm) that are well established in the literature as promoting cardiovascular disease (CVD). The American Heart Association lowered its recommendations for a heart-healthy diet to include no more than 5% to 6% of total calories from saturated fat, which is just the amount found naturally in a vegan diet (one consisting of no animal products).

- Dietary cholesterol: Human bodies produce enough cholesterol for adequate functioning. Although evidence suggests that dietary cholesterol may only be a minor player in elevated serum cholesterol levels, high intakes are linked to increased susceptibility to low-density lipoprotein oxidation, both of which are associated with the promotion of CVD. Dietary cholesterol is found almost exclusively in animal products.

- Antibiotics: The vast majority (70% to 80%) of antibiotics used in the US are given to healthy livestock animals to avoid infections inherent in the types of environments in which they are kept. This is, therefore, the number one contributor to the increasingly virulent antibiotic-resistant infections of the type that sickened 2 million and killed 23,000 Americans in 2013.

- Insulin-like growth factor-1: Insulin like growth factor-1 is a hormone naturally found in animals, including humans. This hormone promotes growth. When insulin-like growth factor-1 is consumed, not only is the added exogenous dose itself taken in, but because the amino acid profile typical of animal protein stimulates the body's production of insulin-like growth factor-1, more is generated endogenously. Fostering growth as a full-grown adult can promote cancer proliferation.

- Heme iron: Although heme iron, found in animal products, is absorbed at a higher rate than nonheme iron, found in plant-based and fortified foods, absorption of nonheme iron can be increased by pairing plant-based protein sources with foods high in vitamin C. Additionally, research suggests that excess iron is pro-oxidative and may increase colorectal cancer risk and promote atherosclerosis and reduced insulin sensitivity.

- Chemical contaminants formed from high temperature cooking of cooked animal products: When flesh is cooked, compounds called polycyclic aromatic hydrocarbons, heterocyclic amines, and advanced glycation end products are formed. These compounds are carcinogenic, pro-inflammatory, prooxidative, and contributive to chronic disease.

- Carnitine: Carnitine, found primarily in meat, may be converted in the body by the gut bacteria to produce trimethylamine N-oxide (TMAO). High levels of trimethylamine n-oxide are associated with inflammation, atherosclerosis, heart attack, stroke, and death.

- N-Glycolylneuraminic acid (Neu5Gc): This compound is found in meat and promotes chronic inflammation.

On the other hand, there are infinite advantages to the vast array of nutrients found in plant foods. Phytochemicals and fibers are the two categories of nutrients that are possibly the most health promoting and disease fighting. Plants are the only source of these nutrients; they are completely absent in animals. Plants contain thousands of phytochemicals, such as carotenoids, glucosinolates, and flavonoids, which perform a multitude of beneficial functions, including:

- Antioxidation, neutralizing free radicals
- Anti-inflammation
- Cancer activity reduction via several mechanisms, including inhibiting tumor growth, detoxifying carcinogens, retarding cell growth, and preventing cancer formation
- Immunity enhancement
- Protection against certain diseases, such as osteoporosis, some cancers, CVD, macular degeneration, and cataracts
- Optimization of serum cholesterol.

Fibers found in whole plant foods powerfully support the gastrointestinal, cardiovascular, and immune systems through multiple mechanisms. Yet more than 90% of adults and children in the US do not get the minimum recommended dietary fiber. Thus, it can be advantageous for physicians to recommend and support plantbased eating to achieve optimal health outcomes and possibly minimize the need for procedures, medications, and other treatments. Aiming for lifestyle changes as primary prevention has been estimated to save upwards of 70% to 80% of health care costs because 75% of health care spending in the US goes to treat people with chronic conditions. Offering this option and guiding patients through the logistics and their concerns about plantbased eating is a viable first line of therapy in the clinical setting. This article will delineate how best to achieve a well-balanced, nutrient-dense meal plan, define notable nutrient sources, describe how to get started, and offer suggestions on how physicians can encourage and work with their patients who are interested to maintain adherence and enjoy success.

NOTABLE NUTRIENTS

Although nutrient deficiency is a primary concern for many people when considering plant-based eating, the Academy of Nutrition and Dietetics states that "vegetarian diets, including total vegetarian or vegan diets, are healthful, nutritionally adequate, and may provide health benefits in the prevention and treatment of certain diseases." The Academy's position paper goes on to conclude that "well-planned vegetarian diets are appropriate for individuals during all stages of the life cycle, including pregnancy, lactation, infancy, childhood, and adolescence, and for athletes." Because any type of meal plan should be approached with careful thought, it is helpful to note that plant-based diets, including calorie-restricted, weight-loss diets, have been found to be more nutritionally sound than typical dietary patterns.

A well-balanced, plant-based diet is composed of vegetables, fruits, whole grains, legumes, herbs, spices, and a small amount of nuts and seeds. Half of the plate should consist of vegetables and fruits in accordance with the US Department of Agriculture, American Cancer Society, and American Heart Association, because they are filled with fiber, potassium, magnesium, iron, folate, and vitamins C and A—almost all of the nutrients that tend to run low in the American population, according to the Scientific Report of the 2015 Dietary Guidelines Advisory Committee. Legumes are excellent sources of lysine (an amino acid that may fall short in a plant-based diet), fiber, calcium, iron, zinc, and selenium. It is ideal to consume one to one-and-a-half cups of legumes per day. Substantiating meals with whole grains aids with satiety, energy, and versatility in cuisine.

Nuts are nutritional nuggets, brimming with essential fats, protein, fiber, vitamin E, and plant sterols, and have been shown to promote cardiovascular health and protect against type 2 diabetes and obesity, macular degeneration, and cholelithiasis. One oz to 2 oz (or 30 g to 60 g) of nuts per day is recommended. Seeds, too, are special in that their essential fat ratios are well-balanced, and they contain multiple trace minerals and phytochemicals. One or 2 tablespoons per day will boost overall nutrition. Opting for whole food sources of fats, as opposed to extracted fats as found in oils, is optimal to decrease caloric density and increase nutrient and fiber consumption. Herbs and spices also contain phytochemicals and help make food delicious, varied, and exciting, and should be used according to preference.

PLANT-BASED MACRONUTRITION

All calories (kcals) come from some combination of carbohydrates (4 kcals/g), proteins (4 kcals/g), and fats (9 kcals/g). Alcohol also provides calories (7 kcals/g) but is not considered an essential nutrient. The ideal ratio of intake of these 3 macronutrients is highly controversial and debatable. There is plenty of evidence supporting health and weight management benefits of low-fat/high-carbohydrate diets, as seen in the traditional Okinawan diet and in Dean Ornish, MD's and Caldwell Esselstyn, MD's reversal of advanced coronary artery disease and Neal Barnard, MD's reduction of glycemia in type 2 diabetes using a plant-based diet with 10% of calories from fat.

Similarly, the Mediterranean and many raw food diets consisting of upwards of 36% or more of calories from fat show consistently positive health advantages. Thus, it appears that it is likely the quality of the diet that is responsible for health outcomes rather than the ratio of macronutrients.

Carbohydrates

The Institute of Medicine's adequate intake of carbohydrates is 130 g/d for everyone (except during pregnancy and lactation) beginning at age 1 year. Optimal sources of carbohydrates, such as wholesome vegetables, fruits, whole grains, and legumes, are high in fiber and nutrients. Refined carbohydrates from sugars, flours, and other processed foods can lead to malnourishment and promote illness.

Protein

Adequate intake of protein is based on weight and is estimated at 1.5 g/kg/d for infants, 1.1 g/kg/d for 1 to 3 year olds, 0.95 g/kg/d for 4 to 13 year olds, 0.85 g/kg/d for 14 to 18 year olds, 0.8 g/kg/d for adults, and 1.1 g/kg/d for pregnant (using prepregnancy weight) and lactating women. Protein is readily available throughout the plant kingdom, but those foods that are particularly rich in protein include legumes, nuts and nut butters, seeds and seed butters, soy foods, and intact whole grains.

Fats

Fats—or fatty acids—are more complicated because there are several different chemical varieties based on level and type of saturation. Each category of fatty acid performs different functions and acts uniquely in the body. The essential fatty acids are polyunsaturated and include both omega-3 and omega-6 fatty acids. Omega-3 fats are found in their shorter chain form as alpha linolenic acid and are used as energy. They are also converted by the body to the longer-chain eicosapentaenoic acid (EPA) and then docosahexaenoic acid (DHA). Because this conversion process can be inefficient, some people may require a direct source of these longerchain EPA and DHA in the form of a microalgae supplement.

Alpha linolenic acid can be found in flaxseeds, hempseeds, chia seeds, leafy green vegetables (both terrestrial and marine), soybeans and soy products, walnuts, and wheat germ, as well as in their respective oils. A direct plant source of EPA and DHA is microalgae, through which fish acquire them. Plant sources may be superior because they do not contain the contaminants that fish contain, including heavy metals, such as mercury, lead, and cadmium, as well as industrial pollutants. Also, plant sources are more sustainable than fish sources. Monounsaturated fats are not essential but have been found to impart either a neutral or slightly beneficial effect on serum cholesterol levels, depending on which nutrient they are replacing. When swapped for saturated fats, trans fats, or refined carbohydrates, monounsaturated fats may lower low-density lipoprotein and raise high-density lipoprotein cholesterol.

These fatty acids are found in olives, avocados, macadamia nuts, hazelnuts, pecans, peanuts, and their respective oils, as well as in canola, sunflower, and safflower oils. Saturated fats, as mentioned above, are not essential in the diet and can promote CVD. They are found primarily in animal products but are available in some plant foods, mostly in tropical fats and oils, such as palm and coconut, and also in other high-fat foods, including avocados, olives, nuts, and seeds. If a vegan diet contains an average of 5% to 6% of kcals from saturated fat, which is what the American Heart Organization recommends for a heart-healthy diet, any added serving of animal products will significantly increase the total intake. Trans fatty acids are laboratory-made via hydrogenation and are found in processed, fried, and fast foods. Although they were originally developed to be a healthy alternative to butter and lard, trans fatty acids were found to significantly increase CVD risk.

In November 2013, the US Food and Drug Administration issued a notice that trans fatty acids were no longer considered safe and is now trying to eliminate artificially produced trans fatty acids (there are small amounts found naturally in meat and dairy products) from the food supply. Be aware that a nutritional label can state a food product contains "0 g trans fats" even if it contains up to 0.5 g per serving. Thus, advise your patients to focus on the ingredient list on food products and to avoid anything with the words "partially hydrogenated." Dietary cholesterol is a sterol that is found primarily in animal products. Although cholesterol is required for the production of hormones, vitamin D, and bile acids, the liver produces enough cholesterol on its own. Excessive intake of dietary cholesterol is associated with increased risk of CVD. Phytosterols, which are similar to cholesterol, are plant-based sterols found in all plant foods (especially wheat germ, nuts, seeds, whole grains, legumes, and unrefined plant oils). Phytosterols reduce cholesterol absorption in the gut, thereby optimizing lipid profiles.

Together with viscous fibers, soy proteins, and almonds, phytosterols have been found to be as effective as statins in some studies in lowering low-density lipoprotein cholesterol. It is crucial to note that all whole foods contain all three macronutrients. It is a pervasive misunderstanding to identify a food as a "carb," "protein," or "fat." Instead, these are all nutrients within a complex of other myriad constituents that are beyond the oversimplification perpetuated by the media and trendy diet fads. Ideally, a healthful diet is loaded with wholesome carbohydrates, moderate in fat, and temperate in protein. The emphasis must be on the quality of the totality of foods coming from whole plant sources as opposed to calculations and perfect ratios.

PLANT-BASED MICRONUTRITION

All nutrients, with the exception of vitamin B12 and possibly vitamin D, which is ideally sourced from the skin's exposure to the sun's ultraviolet rays, can be found in plants. They are also packaged together with thousands of powerful disease-fighting nutrients that work synergistically to support optimal health.

Vitamin B12

Cobalamin, commonly referred to as vitamin B12, is the only nutrient not directly available from plants. This is because vitamin B12 is synthesized by microorganisms, bacteria, fungi, and algae, but not by plants or animals. Animals consume these microorganisms along with their food, which is why this vitamin can be found in their meat, organs, and byproducts (eggs and dairy). Vitamin B12 deficiency can lead to irreversible neurologic disorders, gastrointestinal problems, and megaloblastic anemia. Among other populations, vegans who do not supplement with a reliable source of vitamin B12 or breastfeeding infants of vegan mothers who are not consuming a regular reliable source of vitamin B12 are at risk for deficiency. The body can store vitamin B12 for approximately three to five years, but after that, with no repletion or with inability to absorb, deficiency symptoms may present; deficiency may also be asymptomatic. Because of this lag time and because serum tests for B12 levels can be skewed by other variables, irreversible damage may occur before a deficiency is caught. In a vegan diet, vitamin B12 can be found in fortified plant milks, cereals, or nutritional yeast. However, these are not dependable means of achieving B12 requirements.

Although there are claims that fermented foods, spirulina, chlorella, certain mushrooms, and sea vegetables, among other foods, can provide B12, the vitamin is not usually biologically active. These inactive forms act as B12 analogues, attaching to B12 receptors, preventing absorption of the functional version, and thereby promoting deficiency. The most reliable method of avoiding deficiency for vegans or anyone else at risk is to take a B12 supplement. Because the body can absorb only approximately 1.5 µg to 2.0 µg at a time, it is ideal to supplement with a dose greater than the Recommended Dietary Allowance (RDA) to ensure adequate intake. Plant-based nutrition experts recommend a total weekly dose of 2000 µg to 2500 µg. This can be split into daily doses or into 2 to 3 doses of 1000 µg each per week to help enhance absorption. Because vitamin B12 is water soluble, toxicity is rare.

Vitamin D

Vitamin D, or calciferol, is also known as the "sunshine vitamin" because it is the only nutrient that is acquired from the sun. Although vitamin D is classified as and treated like a fat-soluble vitamin, it is actually a prohormone produced in the skin upon exposure to ultraviolet B sun radiation and then activated by the liver and kidneys. Although human bodies evolved to produce vitamin D via the sun, there appears to be a worldwide epidemic of deficiency. Vitamin D is not widely available from the food supply. Sources of preformed vitamin D include fish liver oil, oily fish, liver, and in smaller doses, meat and egg yolk—foods that also contain high concentrations of saturated fat, cholesterol, and other less-than-ideal components. Vitamin D from sunshine and animal sources is in the form of cholecalciferol, or vitamin D3. A second form called ergocalciferol, or vitamin D2, is found in plant sources, mostly in ultraviolet B-irradiated mushrooms.

However, a plant-derived version of D3 made by lichen was recently discovered. Dietary supplements may contain either D2 or D3, both of which can be effective at optimizing blood levels. More and more physicians are testing for serum levels of vitamin D using the 25-hydroxyvitamin D test. The Institute of Medicine concluded that adequate serum 25-hydroxyvitamin D levels are ≥ 50 nmol/L (≥ 20 ng/mL). If patients have suboptimal levels, emphasizing food sources (especially fortified plant milks) as well as supplements may be helpful. Dosing may be tricky because of variable responses in individuals and differences in types of vitamin D formulas. Of note, although both of the 2 forms of vitamin D—cholecalciferol (D3) and ergocalciferol (D2)—are effective at raising serum D levels in small doses (4000 IU or less), cholecalciferol (D3) is superior when using large boluses. Because the supplement industry is not regulated by the Food and Drug Administration, it is "buyer beware" in the supplement market. Thus, aim to find well-reputed companies. A few organizations, such as Consumer Lab, NSF International, and US Pharmacopeia, act as independent third parties and offer seals of approval after testing products for potency and contaminants. They do not, however, test for safety or efficacy.

Calcium

Calcium, a macromineral, is the most abundant mineral in the human body. A mere 1% of the body's calcium circulates in the blood and tissues; 99% is stored in the bones and teeth. Calcium is a nutrient of concern for the general population with respect to bone mineral optimization during the lifespan. However, because bone metabolism is multifactorial and complex, it is important to emphasize consumption of ample sources of calcium as well as vitamins K and B12, fluoride, magnesium, phosphorus, and potassium; to maintain serum vitamin D levels; and to ensure consistent exercise. Throughout the lifespan, dietary recommendations for adequate intake of calcium fluctuate.

Excellent plant sources of calcium include leafy green vegetables—especially bok choy, broccoli, napa cabbage, collard greens, dandelion greens, kale, turnip greens, and watercress—as well as fortified plant milks, calcium-set tofu, dried figs, sesame seeds and tahini, tempeh, almonds and almond butter, oranges, sweet potatoes, and beans. No matter how much calcium is consumed, the amount that is actually absorbed is more significant. Many variables affect calcium levels via absorption or excretion, including:

- Overall consumption determines how much is absorbed. Only about 500 mg can be absorbed at a time, and absorption decreases as calcium intake increases

- Age. Calcium absorption peaks in infants and children, as they are rapidly growing bone, and then progressively decreases with age

- Phytates, compounds found in whole grains, beans, seeds, nuts, and wheat bran, can bind with calcium as well as with other minerals and inhibit absorption. Soaking, sprouting, leavening, and fermenting improve absorption

- Oxalates are constituents found in some leafy green vegetables, such as spinach, Swiss chard, collard greens, parsley, leeks, and beet greens; berries; almonds; cashews; peanuts; soybeans; okra; quinoa; cocoa; tea; and chocolate. They may also somewhat inhibit absorption of calcium and other minerals, but some may still be absorbed. Emphasizing variety in the foods eaten on a regular basis encourages adequate absorption

- Serum vitamin D levels must be within optimum range in order for the body to absorb calcium.
- Excessive intake of sodium, protein, caffeine, and phosphorus (as from dark sodas) may enhance calcium excretion.

Iron

Ironically, iron is one of the most abundant metals on Earth and yet iron deficiency is one of the most common and widespread nutritional deficiencies. It is the most common deficiency in the world and is a public health problem in both industrialized and nonindustrialized countries. It is particularly prevalent in women of childbearing age, pregnant women, infants, children, teenage girls, and anyone experiencing bleeding, such as people with ulcers, inflamed intestines caused by malabsorptive disorders, or heavy menstruation. Iron-deficiency anemia is no more common in vegetarians than in nonvegetarians. Because plant-sourced iron is nonheme iron, which is susceptible to compounds that inhibit and enhance its absorption, the recommendation for vegans and vegetarians is to aim for slightly more iron than nonvegetarians. Fortunately, this is easy to do with the wide array of iron-rich food choices in the plant kingdom.

Leafy greens and legumes are excellent sources of iron and a multitude of other nutrients, so it is advantageous to include these foods often. Other good choices include soy products, dark chocolate, blackstrap molasses, sesame seeds, tahini, pumpkin seeds, sunflower seeds, raisins, prunes, and cashews. Iron absorption may be diminished in the presence of phytates, tannic acids from tea, calcium in dairy, fiber, polyphenols in coffee and cocoa, and certain spices (eg, turmeric, coriander, chilies, and tamarind). To minimize this, separate iron-rich foods from these nutrients as much as possible. An example is to drink coffee or tea separately from meals or to mix up meal combinations. One of the best tips for optimizing iron absorption is to eat iron-rich foods in combination with foods high in vitamin C and organic acids. This improves solubility, thereby facilitating absorption. Examples of such optimizing food combinations are a green smoothie with leafy greens (iron) and fruit (vitamin C) or salad greens (iron) with tomatoes (vitamin C).

Iodine

Dietary sources of the trace mineral iodine are unreliable and fluctuate geographically because of varying soil qualities. It is crucial for vegans to be mindful of consuming a source of iodine to avoid thyroid issues. Sources of iodine include iodized salt and sea vegetables. However, it is important to note that iodine is not found in sea salts, gourmet salts, or other salty foods. One half-teaspoon of iodized salt provides the daily recommended 150-µg dose.

Also, iodine levels in sea vegetables fluctuate dramatically, with some (especially dulse and nori) containing safe amounts and others (such as kelp) harboring toxic doses. Hijiki, also spelled hiziki, should be avoided owing to its excessive arsenic levels. A preexisting iodine deficiency, a selenium deficiency, or high intake of goitrogens (antinutrients found in cruciferous vegetables, soy products, flaxseeds, millet, peanuts, peaches, pears, pine nuts, spinach, sweet potatoes, and strawberries) can interfere with iodine absorption. There is no need to avoid goitrogenic foods as long as iodine intake is sufficient. If a patient does not enjoy sea vegetables or is minimizing intake of salt, an iodine supplement may be warranted.

Selenium

Selenium is a potent antioxidant that protects against cellular damage and also plays a role in thyroid hormone regulation, reproduction, and dialpha nucleic acid (DNA) synthesis. Brazil nuts are an especially rich source of selenium in the plant kingdom. Although selenium content varies depending on the source, an average ounce (approximately 6 to 8 nuts) can provide 777% of the RDA. When accessible, one Brazil nut a day is an ideal way of meeting selenium recommendations. Other plant sources include whole grains, legumes, vegetables, seeds, and other nuts.

Zinc

Zinc supports immune function and wound healing; synthesis of protein and DNA; and growth and development throughout pregnancy, childhood, and adolescence. Because of the presence of phytates, bioavailability of zinc from plants is lower than from animal products. Zinc deficiency may be difficult to detect in blood tests but can show up clinically as delayed wound healing, growth retardation, hair loss, diminished immunity, suppressed appetite, taste abnormalities, or skin or eye lesions. Consider advising patients to aim for 50% or greater than the RDA of zinc daily by including legumes, cashews and other nuts, seeds, soy products, and whole grains. Preparation methods such as soaking, sprouting, leavening, and fermenting will improve absorption.

Indian Summer Tuscan Quinoa Salad

(Prep Time: 5 min | Cooking Time: 10 min | Servings 6)

Ingredients:

- 1 can of white beans
- 1 cup of quinoa
- ½ cup of cherry tomato, quartered
- ¼ cup of olive oil
- ¼ cup of red onion, finely chopped
- ¼ cup of red bell pepper, diced
- 2 tablespoons of fresh basil, finely chopped
- 1 ½ tablespoons of fresh lemon juice
- Black pepper
- Salt

Directions:

1. Cook the quinoa according to the directions on the package.

2. Whisk the basil with lemon juice, olive oil, a pinch of salt and pepper in a small bowl to make the dressing.
3. Combine the rest of the ingredients in a large mixing bowl then add the dressing and toss it gently
4. Adjust the seasoning of your salad then serve it right away and enjoy.

Make it tastier:

To make it tastier, add 2 tablespoons of balsamic vinegar to the salad to make it tastier.

(Calories: 429 | Total Fat: 11.7 g | Protein: 20.9 g| Total Carbs: 62.4 g)

Sweet Potato Quinoa Bloom Salad

(Prep Time: 10 min | Cooking Time: 40 min | Servings 4)

Ingredients:

- 4 sweet potato, peeled and diced
- 1 can of black beans, drained
- ½ cup of scallion, sliced
- ½ cup of quinoa
- ½ cup of cilantro, finely chopped
- 4 tablespoons of olive oil
- 1 tablespoon of lime juice
- 1 teaspoon of cumin seeds
- 2 teaspoon of paprika
- 2 cloves of garlic, minced
- The zest of 1 lemon
- Black pepper
- Salt

Directions:

1. Preheat the oven on 425 F.

2. Toss 1 teaspoon of paprika with the sweet potato and 1 tablespoon of olive oil in a large bowl then spread it on a lined baking sheet.
3. Bake the potatoes for 20 min then stir it and bake it for another 20 min.
4. Combine 1 teaspoon of paprika with raw quinoa and lemon zest in a heated pot then stir into it 2 cups of water and bring it to a boil.
5. Add a pinch of salt to the quinoa and simmer it for 15 to 20 min.
6. Whisk the rest of the olive oil with garlic and lime juice in a small bow to make the dressing.
7. Combine the rest of the ingredients in a large bowl and stir into it the dressing.
8. Adjust the seasoning of the salad then serve it and enjoy.

Make it tastier:

To make it tastier add in 1 cup of halved cherry tomatoes to the salad then serve
it and enjoy.

(Calories: 393 | Total Fat: 17 g | Protein: 5.7 g| Total Carbs: 56.9 g)

Club Vizia Cucumber Summer Salad

(Prep Time: 10 min | Cooking Time: 0 min | Servings 4)

Ingredients:

- 6 tomatoes, diced
- 2 avocados, peeled and diced
- 2 cucumbers, peeled and diced
- 1 cup of cilantro, finely chopped
- 3 tablespoons of fresh lime juice
- 1 tablespoon of olive oil
- ¼ teaspoon of spike seasoning
- Salt

Directions:

1. Whisk the spike seasoning with olive oil and 2 tablespoons of lime juice in a small bowl to make the dressing.

2. Combine the avocado with 1 tablespoon of lime juice and a pinch of salt in a small bowl.
3. Combine the rest of the ingredients, dressing and the avocado in a large bowl and adjust their seasoning.
4. Adjust the seasoning of your salad then serve it right away and enjoy.

Make it tastier:

To make it tastier, add 1 tablespoon of freshly chopped oregano with basil and enjoy.

(Calories: 292 | Total Fat: 23.7 g | Protein: 4.6 g| Total Carbs: 21.4 g)

Cambria Chickpea Potato Salad

(Prep Time: 5 min | Cooking Time: 25 min | Servings 2 to 3)

Ingredients:

- 1 large sweet potato, peeled and diced
- 1 can of chickpeas, drained
- ½ red onion, finely chopped
- 1 handful of fresh parsley, finely chopped
- 2 tablespoons of fresh lemon juice
- 1 tablespoon of olive oil
- 2 teaspoons of cumin
- 2 cloves of garlic, peeled and minced
- 1 teaspoon of ground coriander
- ½ teaspoon of cayenne pepper
- Black pepper
- Salt

1. Directions:

2. Heat the oil in a pan and sauté in it the sweet potato from all sides.
3. Season the potato with 1 teaspoon of cumin, a pinch of salt and pepper.
4. Toss the sweet potato with the rest of the ingredients in a large bowl then adjust its seasoning.
5. Serve your salad right away and enjoy.

Make it tastier:

To make it tastier, add in ½ cup of corn and 2 tablespoons of freshly chopped dill to the salad and enjoy.

(Calories: 607| Total Fat: 13.7 g | Protein: 28.7 g| Total Carbs: 97 g)

Oasis Fresh Spring Rainbow Salad

(Prep Time: 10 min | Cooking Time: 0 min | Servings 4)

Ingredients:

Dressing:

- 1/3 cup of silken tofu
- 1/3 cup of olive oil
- ¼ white onion, finely chopped
- ¼ cup of vegan mayonnaise
- ¼ cup of apple cider vinegar
- 1 tablespoon of blue poppy seeds
- 1 tablespoon of agave nectar
- 1 tablespoon of nutritional yeast
- 1 teaspoon of mustard

Salad:

- 8 ounces of pasta, cooked
- 1 small cucumber, peeled and diced

- 1 cup of edamame beans
- ½ cup of red cabbage, shredded
- 2 small carrots, diced
- 3 radishes, diced
- ½ yellow bell pepper, seeded and diced
- 1 small golden beet, peeled and diced
- Salt

Directions:

1. Combine all the dressing ingredients in a food processor and blend them smooth.
2. Combine all the salad ingredients in a large bowl and add to it the dressing then toss it gently.
3. Chill the salad in the fridge until it is ready to serve and enjoy.

Make it tastier:

To make it tastier, toss in 10 quartered grape tomatoes to the salad and enjoy.

(Calories: 262 | Total Fat: 2.1 g | Protein: 10.6 g| Total Carbs: 53 g)

Viperia Persian Rice Salad

(Prep Time: 5 min | Cooking Time: 2 h 10 min | Servings 2)

Ingredients:

- 2 cups of basmati rice, cooked and cooled down ½ cup of carrots, shredded ¼ cup of smoked almonds
- ¼ cup of golden raisins
- ½ teaspoon of saffron
- 1 pinch of turmeric
- Salt

Directions:

1. Mix the saffron with turmeric, a pinch of salt and cooked rice in a large bowl.
2. Stir in the rest of the ingredients and adjust the seasoning of the salad then serve it and enjoy.

Make it tastier:

To make it tastier, add in ½ cup of chopped dates and cashews to the salad and enjoy.

(Calories: 405| Total Fat: 3.6 g | Protein: 8.3 g| Total Carbs: 83.8 g)

Neutrino Fruity Veggies Salad

(Prep Time: 15 min | Cooking Time: 15 min | Servings 8)

Ingredients:

Dressing:

- 2 tablespoons of red wine vinegar
- 1 tablespoon of maple syrup
- 1 tablespoon of Dijon mustard
- 1 tablespoon of apple cider vinegar
- 1 clove of garlic, minced
- The juice of 1 lemon
- Black pepper
- Salt

Salad:

- 1 cup of red grapes, seedless and halved
- 1 yellow bell pepper, diced
- 1 orange bell pepper, diced

- 1 small cucumber, peeled and diced
- 1 small head of broccoli, finely chopped
- ¼ cup of sunflower seeds, shelled
- ¼ cup of fresh parsley, finely chopped
- Salt

Directions:

1. Combine all the dressing ingredients in a food processor and blend them smooth.
2. Combine all the salad ingredients in a large bowl and add to it the dressing then toss it gently.
3. Chill the salad in the fridge for 1 to 2 h then serve it enjoy.

Make it tastier:

To make it tastier, add in 3 tablespoons fresh dill to the salad and enjoy.

(Calories: 53 | Total Fat: 1.1 g | Protein: 2 g| Total Carbs: 9.8 g)

Mystic Herbed Butternut Squash Bites

(Prep Time: 25 min | Cooking Time: 25 min | Servings 10)

Ingredients:

- 2 to 3 pound of butternut squash, peeled and diced
- 1/3 cup of mixed herbs, finely chopped (thyme, parsley...)
- 4 cloves of garlic, minced
- Black pepper
- Salt

Directions:

1. Fill 1 inch of a saucepan of water and lower in it a steamer basket then fill it with the butternut squash dices.
2. Cover the saucepan and cook the butternut squash for 13 to 15 min.

3. Heat the oil in a skillet and brown in it the garlic for 2 min.
4. Once the time is up, transfer the garlic with oil to a large mixing bowl with the herbs and the cooked butternut squash dices.
5. Stir them gently without mashing the butternut squash then adjust its seasoning.
6. Refrigerate your herbed butternut squash bites until it completely cools down then serve it and enjoy.

Make it tastier:

To make it tastier, add in ½ teaspoon of dry Italian seasoning to the butternut with the rest of the herbs.

(Calories: 69 | Total Fat: 0.4 g | Protein: 1.5 g| Total Carbs: 17.5 g)

Chevre Roasted Baby Potatoes

(Prep Time: 10 min | Cooking Time: 35 min | Servings 4)

Ingredients:

- 1 ½ pound of baby potatoes, rinsed and halved
- 2 cloves of garlic, peeled and minced
- ½ teaspoon of lemon juice
- ½ teaspoon of dry oregano
- Olive oil
- Black pepper
- Salt

Directions:

1. Preheat the oven on 425 F.
2. Toss the potatoes with the rest of the ingredients in a large bowl then spread it on a lined up baking sheet.
3. Bake the potatoes for 25 min.

4. Once the time is up, stir the potato and rearrange it then bake it for another 10 min.
5. Serve your roasted potatoes warm and enjoy.

Make it tastier:

To make it tastier, add 1 teaspoon of dry thyme to the potatoes before cooking it.

(Calories: 102 | Total Fat: 0.2 g | Protein: 4.5 g| Total Carbs: 22 g)

Banjo Cabbage Steaks with Tahini Sauce

(Prep Time: 5 min | Cooking Time: 25 min | Servings 2)

Ingredients:

- 1 small head of cabbage, cut into 1 inch steak
- 6 tablespoons of coconut milk
- 4 tablespoons of tahini
- 2 tablespoons of dijon mustard
- 2 tablespoons of olive oil
- 1 tablespoon of lime juice
- 1 clove of garlic
- Black pepper
- Salt

Directions:

1. Preheat the oven on 400 F.

2. Rub the cabbage steaks with the clove of garlic then brush them with 1 tablespoon of olive oil.
3. Lay the cabbage steak on a lined up baking sheet and season them with some salt and pepper then bake them for 20 to 25 min.
4. Once the time is up, allow the cabbage steaks to cool down.
5. Combine the rest of the ingredients in a food processor and blend them smooth to make the tahini sauce.
6. Serve your cabbage steaks with the tahini sauce and enjoy.

Make it tastier:

To make it tastier, add 1 tablespoon of peanut butter to the tahini sauce and enjoy.

(Calories: 176 | Total Fat: 14 g | Protein: 4.2 g| Total Carbs: 12.2 g)

La Concuna Olives Spread

(Prep Time: 5 min | Cooking Time: 0 min |
Servings 2 cups)

Ingredients:

- 10 ounces of kalamata olives, pitted
- 10 ounces of green olives, pitted
- ½ cup of sundried tomato, finely chopped ¼ cup of parsley, finely chopped 2 tablespoons of capers
- 2 tablespoons of olive oil
- 1 tablespoon of lemon zest
- 1 tablespoon of lemon juice
- 2 cloves of garlic, minced

Directions:

1. Combine all the ingredients in a food processor and blend them smooth.
2. Serve your spread with some bread slices and enjoy.

Make it tastier:

To make it tastier, rub the bread slices with some garlic and brush them with the oil then roast them in the oven for 2 to 3 min.
Serve your bread slices with the olives spread and enjoy.

(Calories: 411 | Total Fat: 39.1 g | Protein: 3.3 g| Total Carbs: 19.5 g)

Achilles Winter Quinoa Soup

(Prep Time: 15 min | Cooking Time: 6 h |
Servings 4)

Ingredients:

- 3 cups of water
- 3 cups of veggies broth
- 2 cups of kale, roughly chopped
- 2 cup of cauliflower florets
- 1 cup of sweet potato, peeled and diced
- ½ cup of quinoa, uncooked
- ½ cup of mushroom, sliced
- 2 carrots, halved and sliced
- ½ yellow onion, finely chopped
- 1 tablespoon of coconut oil
- 3 cloves of garlic, peeled and minced
- 1 teaspoon of apple cider vinegar
- 1 teaspoon of black pepper
- 1 teaspoon of dry oregano
- ¼ teaspoon of dry marjoram
- Salt

Directions:

1. Heat the oil in a slow cooker then sauté in it the garlic with onion for 3 min.
2. Add in the carrots with mushroom and cook them for 5 to 10 min then stir in the rest of the ingredients except for the kale.
3. Cover the slow cooker and cook the soup for 6 h on low.
4. Once the time is up, stir in the kale and adjust the seasoning of the soup then cook it for another 30 min.
5. Serve your soup warm and enjoy.

Make it tastier:

To make it tastier, add in ½ cup of corn kernels to the soup then cook it according to the directions above and enjoy.

(Calories: 212| Total Fat: 3 g | Protein: 10.6 g| Total Carbs: 36.9 g)

Quiza Black Bean and Quinoa Soup

(Prep Time: 10 min | Cooking Time: 25 min | Servings 4)

Ingredients:

- 20 ounces of canned black beans, rinsed
- 5 cups of veggies broth
- 3 cups of pumpkin, peeled and diced
- ½ cup of quinoa
- 1 onion, diced
- 5 cloves of garlic, peeled and minced
- 1 tablespoon of olive oil
- 2 bay leaves
- 1 red chili pepper, seeded and diced
- 1 teaspoon of cumin
- ½ teaspoon of dry oregano
- Black pepper
- Salt

Directions:

1. Heat the oil in a pot and sauté in it the onion for 3 min then stir in the chili pepper with garlic and cook them for 1 min.
2. Stir in the pumpkin dices with oregano, cumin and bay leaves then cook them for 2 min.
3. Add in the quinoa with 2 cups of broth and bring the soup to a boil then simmer it for 5 min.
4. Once the time is up, stir in the rest of the ingredients and bring the soup to a boil again then simmer it for 10 min.
5. Adjust the seasoning of your soup then serve it warm and enjoy.

Make it tastier:

To make it tastier, stir in ½ cup of creamy peanut butter once it is done then serve it warm and enjoy.

(Calories: 722 | Total Fat: 9.2 g | Protein: 42.4 g| Total Carbs: 122.3 g)

Le Vin Vegan Moroccan Harira (Soup)

(Prep Time: 15 min | Cooking Time: 45 min | Servings 4)

Ingredients:

- 28 ounces of fresh tomato, crushed
- 6 cups of veggies broth
- 2 cups of onions, peeled and finely chopped
- 2 carrots, peeled and sliced
- 1 ½ cups of dry red lentils
- 1/3 cup of cilantro, finely chopped
- 1/3 cup of parsley, finely chopped
- 1 ½ teaspoons of cumin
- ¾ teaspoon of ground ginger
- ¾ teaspoon of paprika
- ¾ teaspoon of cinnamon powder
- ¾ teaspoon of cumin
- ¾ teaspoon of turmeric powder
- The juice of 1 lemon
- 2 cloves of garlic, peeled and minced
- Black pepper

- Salt

Directions:

1. Heat ¼ cup of the broth in a large pot then sauté in it the onion with carrot and garlic for 3 to 5 min.
2. Add the cumin with turmeric, ginger, paprika and cinnamon then cook them for another minute.
3. Once the time is up, stir in the rest of the ingredients and cover the pot then bring it to a boil then simmer it for 35 min on low heat.
4. Adjust the seasoning of the soup then serve it warm and enjoy.

Make it faster:

To reduce 5 min of the cooking process, substitute the fresh tomato with canned tomato and enjoy.

(Calories: 391 | Total Fat: 3.6 g | Protein: 28.8 g| Total Carbs: 62.1 g)

Bluez Creamy Purple Soup

(Prep Time: 5 min | Cooking Time: 5 min |
Servings 2 to 4)

Ingredients:

- 2 cans of black beans
- 1 ½ cups of water
- 2 carrots, finely chopped
- ½ red bell pepper, seeded and diced
- 2 stalks of celery, diced
- ½ white onion, finely chopped
- 2 cloves of garlic, minced
- 1 teaspoon of cumin powder
- Black pepper
- Salt

Directions:

1. Combine all the ingredients in a food processor and blend them smooth.

2. Transfer the soup to a saucepan and simmer it for 5 min.
3. Adjust the seasoning of your soup then serve it warm and enjoy.

Make it tastier:

To make it tastier, stir in 1 ½ tablespoons of lemon juice when it is done then serve it warm and enjoy.

(Calories: 753 | Total Fat: 3.2 g | Protein: 46.7 g| Total Carbs: 138 g)

Tivondra Tasty Chaos Soup

(Prep Time: 5 min | Cooking Time: 2 h 10 min | Servings 6)

Ingredients:

- 14 ounces of coconut milk
- 10.5 ounces of rice noodles
- 8 ounces of tofu, sliced
- 5 cups of veggies broth
- 1 cup of mushroom, sliced
- 1 cup of bean sprouts
- ¼ cup of cilantro leaves
- ¼ cup of basil leaves
- 1 small bunch of green onions, finely chopped
- 1 inch of fresh ginger, peeled and sliced
- 2 tablespoons of curry paste
- 5 kaffir lime leaves
- The juice of ½ lime
- Salt

Directions:

1. Combine the broth with coconut milk in a pot and bring them to a simmer then stir in the curry paste until it dissolves.
2. Add in the mushroom with basil, cilantro and lime leaves, green onions and rice noodles then simmer the soup for 5 min.
3. Once the time is up, stir in the bean sprouts and simmer the soup for another minute.
4. Add in the tofu slices with a pinch of salt and pepper then serve your soup right away and enjoy.

Make it tastier:

To make it tastier, stir in ¼ cup of corn kernels to the soup with the mushroom...

(Calories: 290 | Total Fat: 20.8 g | Protein: 7.8 g| Total Carbs: 21.6 g)

Plethora Garlicky Eggplant Casserole

(Prep Time: 10 min | Cooking Time: 1 h |
Servings 4)

Ingredients:

- 2 large eggplants, sliced
- 3 tomatoes, sliced
- 1 cup of water
- 2 tablespoon of tomato paste
- ½ teaspoon of garlic powder
- ½ teaspoon of dry thyme
- ½ teaspoon of dry basil
- Black pepper
- Salt
- Vegetable oil

Directions:

1. Heat some vegetable oil in a pan the fry in it the eggplant slices for 3 min on each side then drain them and set them aside.

2. Combine the tomato with water, garlic, thyme, basil, a pinch of salt and pepper in a saucepan until the tomato paste dissolves.
3. Bring the water boil to a boil then turn off the heat and set it aside.
4. Preheat the oven on 400 F.
5. Grease a baking dish with some olive oil then layer in it the eggplant and tomato slices.
6. Pour the water mix all over the eggplant and tomato mix then bake it for 40 min.
7. Once the time is up, serve your eggplant casserole warm and enjoy.

Make it tastier:

To make it tastier, add in 10 ounces of sliced mushroom to the eggplant casserole before cooking it and enjoy.

(Calories: 93 | Total Fat: 0.7 g | Protein: 3.9 g| Total Carbs: 21.5 g)

Bravo Vegan Lasagna

(Prep Time: 5 min | Cooking Time: 1 h 30 min |
Servings 8 to 12)

Ingredients:

Sauce:

- 28 ounces of canned tomatoes, peeled
- 1 yellow onion, finely chopped
- ¼ cup of olive oil
- 2 tablespoons of capers
- 1 tablespoon of tomato paste
- 2 cloves of garlic, peeled and minced
- 1 bay leaf
- Salt

Filling:

- 2 pounds of tofu, drained
- 1 ½ pounds of eggplant, sliced
- 12 ounces of dry vegan lasagna noodles

- 3 tablespoons of nutritional yeast
- 2 tablespoons of fresh lemon juice
- 1 teaspoon of fresh parsley, finely chopped
  Kosher Salt

Directions:

1. Preheat the oven on 350 F.
2. Lay the eggplant slices on 2 lined up baking sheets and sprinkle on them 1 teaspoon of salt then flip them and sprinkle on them another teaspoon of salt.
3. Set the eggplant slices aside and allow them to set for 30 min.
4. Pulse the tomato in a food processor few times until it becomes finely chopped.
5. Heat ¼ cup of olive oil in a saucepan and cook in it the onion for 3 min then stir in the garlic and cook them for another 30 sec.
6. Push the tomato to one side of the saucepan then place the tomato paste in the other side then cook it for 1 min.

7. Once the time is up, stir in the rest of the sauce ingredients and stir them then simmer them on low heat for 45 min.

8. Pat the eggplant slices dry with some paper towels then heat ½ teaspoon of oil in a pan and sear in it the eggplants on batches while adding more oil if needed.

9. Bring a salted pot of water to a boil then cook in it the pasta for 7 min.

10. Combine the rest of the filling ingredients in a food processor and blend them smooth.

11. Spread some of the tomato sauce in the bottom of a baking dish then top it with a layer of pasta followed by 1 cup of the tofu mix, ¼ of the eggplant slices and 1 cup of the tomato sauce.

12. Repeat the process with the rest of the ingredients covering the top of lasagna with some sauce then cover it with a paper foil.

13. Bake the lasagna for 50 min then remove the foil and bake it for 10 min.

14.   Once the time is up, allow the lasagna to cool down for 10 then serve it warm and enjoy.

Make it tastier:

To make it tastier, add in layers of fresh basil leaves on top of every eggplant layer and enjoy.

(Calories: 316 | Total Fat: 12.4 g | Protein: 18 g|
Total Carbs: 38 g)

Speakeasy Mango and Tofu Casserole

(Prep Time: 20 min | Cooking Time: 45 min | Servings 4)

Ingredients:

- 14 ounces of firm tofu, thickly sliced
- 1 ½ cup of coconut milk
- ¾ cup of ripe mango purée
- ¾ cup of red onion, finely chopped
- 4 cloves
- 3 cloves of garlic, peeled and finely chopped
- 2 tablespoons of water
- 3 teaspoons of sunflower oil
- 2 teaspoons of apple cider vinegar
- ½ teaspoon of Garam Masala
- ¼ teaspoon of cumin seeds
- ¼ teaspoon of cinnamon powder
- ¼ teaspoon of cayenne pepper
- Salt

Directions:

1. Cover the tofu with a towel and place on it something that weighs 10 pounds then let it stand for 10 min.
2. Heat 2 teaspoons of oil in a skillet then cut the tofu into dices and brown it in it for 4 min on each side.
3. Stir in the garam masala with cinnamon and cayenne pepper then cook it for 2 min and set it aside.
4. Combine the garlic with onion and water in a food processor then set them aside.
5. Heat the rest of the oil in a pot and cook in it the cloves with cumin seeds for 1 min then stir in the onion purée.
6. Cook the onion purée for 15 min on low heat while stirring it often then stir into it the rest of the ingredients.
7. Cover the pot and cook it for 15 min on low heat then uncover the pot and cook it for another 15 min.
8. Once the time is up, serve your mango tofu casserole warm and

9. enjoy.

Make it tastier:

To make it tastier, stir in ½ cup of chickpeas with the mango, tofu...to you stew before cooking it.

(Calories: 321 | Total Fat: 29.2 g | Protein: 10.6 g| Total Carbs: 9.6 g)

Salud Pasta and Peas Salad

(Prep Time: 5 min | Cooking Time: 12 min |
Servings 4)

Ingredients:

- 1 pound of snow peas, shelled
- 1 pound of fava bean
- 12 ounces of vegan pasta
- ½ cup of water
- ½ cup of cashews, soaked for 4 to 12 h
- 2 tablespoons of lemon juice
- 1 tablespoon of olive oil
- ¼ teaspoon of Dijon mustard

Directions:

1. Combine the mustard with cashews, water, olive oil and lemon juice in a food processor then blend them smooth to make the sauce.

2. Cook the pasta according to the directions on the package.
3. Bring a salted pot of water to a boil and cook in it the fava beans for 2 min then drain it and transfer it directly to a filled bowl with icy water.
4. Shell the fava beans then set them aside.
5. Bring a saltedd pot of water to a boil and cook in it the peas for 1 min 30 sec then drain them and set them aside.
6. Once the time is up, combine the sauce with pasta, fava beans and peas in a large mixing bowl then toss them gently.
7. Serve your pasta and enjoy.

Make it tastier:

To make it tastier, add 1 tablespoon of white miso to the sauce and enjoy.

(Calories: 565 | Total Fat: 13.5 g | Protein: 36 g| Total Carbs: 79.9 g)

Dervish Orangy Chocolate Tart

(Prep Time: 20 min | Cooking Time: 0 min | Servings 6 to 8)

Ingredients:

- 3 cup of cashews, soaked
- 1 cup of fresh orange juice
- 1 cup of whole almonds
- 1 cup of coconut oil, liquid
- ½ cup of dates, pitted and chopped
- ½ cup and ¼ cup of cocoa powder
- ¾ cup of agave nectar
- 1 teaspoon of orange zest, grated

Directions:

1. Combine ¼ cup of cocoa powder with almonds and dates in a food processor then blend them smooth.

2. Grease a springform pan with some coconut oil then pour in it the cocoa mix and pat it to make the crust.
3. Combine the rest of the ingredients in a food processor and blend them smooth for 3 min to make the filling.
4. Pour the filling right on the crust then cover it with foil.
5. Freeze the tart for 8 h then transfer it to a fridge for 1h 30 min.
6. Once the time is up, serve your tart right away and enjoy.

Make it tastier:

To make it tastier, add ¼ teaspoon of mixed nutmeg powder with cinnamon to the crust mix before blending it.

(Calories: 631 | Total Fat: 44.5 g | Protein: 12.1 g| Total Carbs: 27 g)

Conscious Sweet Potato Cake

(Prep Time: 15 min | Cooking Time: 23 min | Servings 6 to 8)

Ingredients:

- 1 cup of purpose flour
- ¾ cup of sweet potato, cooked and peeled ½ cup and 1 tablespoon of water 1/3 cup of coconut sugar
- ¼ cup of maple syrup
- ¼ cup of cocoa powder
- ¼ cup of mini vegan chocolate chips
- 1 tablespoon of balsamic vinegar
- 1 teaspoon of baking soda
- 1 teaspoon of baking powder
- 1 pinch of salt

Directions:

1. Preheat the oven on 350 F.

2. Combine the sweet potato with maple syrup, balsamic vinegar, ½ cup of water and the vanilla extract in a food processor then blend them smooth.

3. Combine the rest of the ingredients in a large bowl then add to them the potato mix and mix them with a fork until they become smooth.

4. Grease a cake pan and line it with a parchment paper then bake it for 21 to 23 min.

5. Once the time is up, allow the cake to cool down completely then serve it and enjoy.

Make it tastier:

To make it tastier, add 2 teaspoons of vanilla extract to the potato mix before blending it.

(Calories: 255 | Total Fat: 2.8 g | Protein: 3.8 g| Total Carbs: 47.4 g)

Mondo Bocci Banana Mousse

(Prep Time: 15 min | Cooking Time: 0 min |
Servings 2)

Ingredients:

- 2 large bananas, mashed
- 1 cup of tofu, whipped
- ½ cup of vegan dark chocolate, melted
- ¼ cup of flaxseed, ground
- 5 tablespoons of water

Directions:

1. Mix the flaxseed with water in a small bowl then let it set for 5 min.
2. Whip the tofu in a large mixing bowl then add to it the rest of the ingredients and whip them again until they become cream.
3. Pipe the mousse into serving glasses then serve them and enjoy.

Make it tastier:

To make it tastier, add 1/8 teaspoon of vanilla extract to the mousse before whipping it.

(Calories: 158 | Total Fat: 6 g | Protein: 5 g| Total Carbs: 23 g)

Bovine Vanilla Ice Cream with Cookie Dough

(Prep Time: 2 h | Cooking Time: 2 h 10 min | Servings 2)

Ingredients:

Ice Cream:

- 14 ounces of coconut milk
- 1 ¼ cup of cashews, soaked for an overnight and drained
- ¼ cup of maple syrup
- ¼ cup of brown sugar
- 2 ½ tablespoons of coconut oil liquid
- 1 teaspoon of vanilla extract

Cookie Dough:

- ½ cup of brown sugar
- ½ cup of creamy and crunchy peanut butter ¾ cup of purpose flour

- ¼ cup of vegan mini chocolate chips
- 3 tablespoons of vegan butter
- 2 tablespoons of coconut milk
- 1 teaspoon of vanilla extract

Directions:

1. Combine all the ice cream ingredients in a food processor and blend them smooth until they become cream.
2. Transfer the mix to a bowl and freeze it for 2 h to an overnight.
3. In the meantime, combine the cookie dough in a bowl and stir them gently then chill it in the fridge until the ice cream is done.
4. Once the time is up, crumble the cookie dough all over the ice cream and freeze it for another 4 h then serve it and enjoy.

Make it tastier:

To make it tastier, stir in ¼ cup of macadamia nuts to the ice cream afterblending it then freeze it and enjoy.

(Calories: 542 | Total Fat: 36 g | Protein: 9.7 g| Total Carbs: 47 g)

Aglaya Vegan Chocolate Cream Drink

(Prep Time: 10 min | Cooking Time: 5 min | Servings 2 to 4)

Ingredients:

5 ounces of vegan dark chocolate

2 cups of coconut milk

1 tablespoon of coconut sugar

½ teaspoon of cinnamon powder

1 pinch of nutmeg powder

1 pinch of salt

Directions:

1. Pour the milk in a saucepan and bring it to pressure then stir into it the chocolate and whisk it until the chocolate completely melts.
2. Whisk in the rest of the ingredients then add in more sugar if you want.

3. Serve your chocolate cream drinks warm
and enjoy.

Make it tastier:

To make it tastier, add in ½ teaspoon of vanilla extract to your chocolate right before serving it and enjoy.

(Calories: 338 | Total Fat: 25 g | Protein: 4.3 g|
Total Carbs: 24 g)

Vegan Shopping List

Introduction

I have learned a lot about plant-based shopping since I became vegan. Many hits and many misses. Hopefully, this vegan shopping list will help you avoid the mistakes I made. My best advice would be to keep it simple, and always have some cooked whole grains, veggies and beans on hand for quick and delicious meals.

I try to stay away from all processed foods, but when I can't avoid it, I read the ingredients carefully. It may say "natural" on the front, but that doesn't mean it's organic or non-GMO. It is particularly important that you avoid all GMO products which have been genetically altered and could be filled with pesticides. So let's get started.

MILK SUBSTITUTES

Any unsweetened organic, non-dairy milk like rice, almond, hemp, cashew, oat, or soy milk. I like almond and soy milk the best.

Hemp milk is a complete protein meaning that it contains all of the amino acids necessary foroptimal health. A single serving of hemp milk provides an entire day's recommended intake of omega 3 fats. It has a nice, light taste and can be added to cereals, oatmeal, smoothies or to drink on its own.

Soy milk has a nutrition profile most similar to dairy milk. It is the highest in protein providingbetween 8 and 11 grams of protein per cup. Tastes great in coffee and dissolves well.

Almond milk tends to be lower in calories and sugar than most non-dairy milk. It also containsmonounsaturated fats, which are heart healthy fats. Almond milk tends to separate when heated so it may separate in coffee.

Cashew milk is the new kid on the block. It is creamy and sweet but can be high in sugar. Make sureyou go for unsweetened.

Rice milk is non-allergenic. However, it is the lowest in protein and tends to be higher in sugar andcalories. Always use unsweetened.

Oat milk provides fiber as well as protein about 4 grams per serving. However, it is on the higherend in terms of sugar and calories.

Almond, hemp, soy, coconut and rice milk can easily be used in baked goods.

All non-dairy milk are vegan and lactose-free.

There are brands of non-dairy milk that incorporate added fats and sweeteners including cane juice and brown rice syrup. I would avoid these and stick with brands that are unsweetened and include only a few simple ingredients

**Some non-dairy milk are fortified with B12.

Check the label if you are looking for B12 fortified.**

BUTTER SUBSTITUTES

Earth Balance is popular and makes lots of vegan butter options. Please use in moderation becausepart of enjoying a healthy, plant-based diet is letting go of excessive oil.

All oil and vegan butter are processed foods. They are pure fat, and most of the great nutrients and properties of the whole food are extracted in the process of making a whole food an oil. If you have heart disease or worry about heart disease, I would recommend no oil at all. Learn more about oil and degenerative disease from heart specialist, Dr. Caldwell Esselstyn or Dr. John McDougall on youtube.

CHEESE SUBSTITUTES

There are many vegan cheese substitutes on the market but always remember these are processed foods. I prefer nut and homemade vegan cheese. Also, just because it is in the vegan cheese section, don't assume it is vegan. Many rice and soy cheese makers add casein (from cow's) to help the cheese melt.

If you like cheese on popcorn, I highly recommend nutritional yeast. It has a similar salty, nutty taste like parmesan and is delicious sprinkled on popcorn. It is also a great cheese replacement for baked macaroni and cheese.

For pasta, I like to grind up some pine nuts and sprinkle them on top. It adds a creamy and salty taste much like parmesan cheese.

On the commercial side, I think Chao cheese slices by Field Roast taste the best. I also like Miyoko's Kitchen vegan mozzarella.

EGG SUBSTITUTES

There are many commercial egg substitutes on the market. I use Bob's Red Mill. I mainly use egg substitutes for baking. I have tried every vegan egg binder imaginable, and I still haven't found one that can hold a vegan burger together perfectly.

Ground flax seed eggs

My favorite. Makes two eggs - Whisk two tablespoons of ground flax seed with six tablespoons of water until fluffy - put the mixture in the refrigerator for 10 minutes to thicken.

Chia Seed Eggs - Makes one egg - Whisk one tablespoon chia seeds with 3 tablespoons of water -mix & let sit for fifteen minutes

Cornstarch Eggs - Makes one egg - Combine two tablespoons of cornstarch with three tablespoonsof water

Arrowroot Eggs - Makes one egg - Combine two tablespoons of Arrowroot with three tablespoonsof water

Chickpea Flour Eggs - Makes one egg - Whisk three tablespoons of Chickpea flour with threetablespoons of water

Applesauce and Bananas - For 2 eggs - Smash up or blend about a half a banana or 1/4 cup applesauceto use as an egg replacer in baked goods such as muffins, pancakes or yeast-free quick breads.

Tofu -For two eggs - blend 1/4 cup silken tofu until tofu is smooth and creamy.

Aquafaba - Aquafaba is the liquid from cooked chickpeas. Three tablespoons equals 1 egg white.If you are using the aquafaba as a binder, you will need to whip the liquid until foamy, not over whipped, with a hand mixer.

MEAT SUBSTITUTES

I don't eat many faux meats, but I have tried the following and they may help you with your transition but remember the best food you can eat are whole, plant-based foods like grains, legumes, fruits, vegetables, and healthy fats like nuts, seeds, and avocado.

Beyond Meat is a popular meat substitute. It is non-GMO, organic and made from plants, not soy.

They make vegan chicken and crumbles.

Gardein Fresh & Frozen Products - I particularly like the vegan turkey cutlets with gravy, and theyalso have beef strips which work nicely marinated for tacos.

Field Roast Sausages - If you are craving a frankfurter or sausage, I think Field Roast tastes the best.Sweet Earth makes a variety of faux meats including vegan bacon. Their ingredients are mainly vegetables and non-GMO.

SWEETENERS

**Please note all white processed cane sugar is whitened with animal
bone char and isn't vegan - see this link for more information**

Unprocessed Stevia for coffee and tea - check and make sure there is only one ingredient on thelabel and no dextrose.

100% Organic Maple Syrup (my favorite sweetener for recipes) Unsulphured Blackstrap Molasses -Has a low glycemic index and is high in iron and magnesium content.

Zulka - 100% Vegan Sugar - The only sugar with the label "no bone char"and available in most grocery stores

CONDIMENTS

Vegan Mayonnaise - There are many manufacturers of vegan mayonnaise. Once again, usesparingly, it is a processed oil based food.

Non-GMO Ketchup, Mustard - Hundreds of brands. Make sure your ketchup doesn't include high-fructose corn syrup

NUTS, SEEDS & DRIED FRUITS

Nuts are high in protein and can be added to almost any meal. I like slivered almonds on salads, oatmeal or just for snacking. Seeds and dried fruits make a wonderful topping for oatmeal and salads. Hemp seeds, ground flax seeds and chia seeds contain a great balance of omega-6 and omega-3s. Have two tablespoons of hemp, ground flax seeds, or chia seeds every day.

Always buy ground flaxseeds since this particular seed has a hard outer cover, making it more difficult to digest. That only applies to flaxseeds.

VEGETABLES

Buy any and all fresh in-season organic vegetables (more reasonably priced when in season) Eat as many vegetables as you like!

Keep a lot of lemons on hand to squeeze over vegetables and greens.

Buy fresh parsley, cilantro, garlic, ginger and mint when possible for additional flavoring.

Cruciferous vegetables help fight cancer and lung problems. Leafy greens are loaded with nutrients and assist in digestion.

PROTEIN

Lentils, Tofu, Beans, Quinoa, Soy, Chick Peas, Green Peas, Artichokes, Hemp Seeds, Chia Seeds, Oatmeal, Pumpkin Seeds, Hemp Milk, Edamame, Spinach, Black Eyed Peas, Broccoli, Asparagus, Green Beans, Almonds, Spirulina, Tahini, Nutritional Yeast, Peanut Butter, and Amaranth all have high amounts of protein.

There is a vegan protein list in the bonus section of the online course

PLANT-BASED MEAT SUBSTITUTES

Tempeh Is made by deep-frying fermented soybeans. It is commonly sold in flat rectangular piecesabout eight inches long. The chewy consistency makes it an exceptional vegetable protein to use as a mock meat substitute, especially in stews and chili.

There are a number of pre-made tempeh products on the market.

Seitan also called "wheat meat" is derived from the protein portion of wheat. It stands in for meat inmany recipes and works so well that some vegans avoid it because the texture is too "meaty." You can buy various pre-made seitan products. It comes cubed for stews or kabobs or as vegan bacon.

Chickpeas - Although not a meat substitute, chickpeas are definitely a protein substitute and mynumber one protein. Mash them up with a little vegan mayo and sun-dried tomatoes and put them on sliced bread with avocado and sprouts. Add them to soups and salads. Or roast them with a little cayenne pepper as an appetizer. Chickpeas are one of the most versatile plant-based foods you can consume. Chickpeas are one of the most versatile proteins in the plant-based world.

Organic non-GMO tofu - The typical tofu textures are Silken (soft), soft, medium, firm and extra-firm. You can add tofu to pretty much anything. It takes on the flavor you cook it with.

WHOLE GRAINS

Grain is considered to be a whole grain as long as all three original parts – the bran, germ, and endosperm are present in the same proportions as when the grain was growing in the field. My favorite whole grains are quinoa, brown rice, farro, and bulgur.

Quinoa - Quinoa is a grain crop that is grown for its edible seeds. It is pronounced KEEN-wah. Itis basically a "seed" which is prepared and eaten similarly to a grain. There are three types: white, red and black. It has a rich nutrient profile, and one one cup has 8 grams of protein, manganese, magnesium, iron, phosphorus, folate, zinc and copper. Quinoa is gluten-free and usually grown organically. Make sure you purchase non-GMO quinoa. One cup of cooked chickpeas contains 15 grams of protein.

Brown Rice - Brown rice is better for you than white. White rice is refined. Brown rice, unlikewhite rice, still has the side hull and bran. The side hulls and brans are rich in protein, thiamine, calcium, magnesium, selenium, fiber and potassium. There are 5 grams of protein in once cup of cooked brown rice.

Farro

Farro is a healthy whole grain that Italians have been eating for years. Farro is an excellent source of protein, fiber and nutrients like magnesium and iron. It has a nutty, chewy flavor and can serve as the bed for any dish. I also love warm farro with non-dairy milk, a few nuts and drizzled with maple syrup.

A cup of farro has about 8 grams of fiber and 7 grams of protein per 1/4 cup dry. This is greater than either quinoa or brown rice. Although not gluten- free, farro has significantly less gluten than wheat.

Bulgur

Bulgur also contains resistant starch. Resistant starch has been called nature's fat-burning breakthrough because resistant starch is bulky, so it takes up space in your digestive system. Because you can't digest it or absorb it, the starch never enters your bloodstream. That means it avoids

the issue of some carbs which can get socked away as body fat when you eat more than you burn. I recommend a cup of bulgur or barley every day for weight loss. Barley, Millet, Teff, Wild Rice, Wheat, Buckwheat, Amaranth, Buckwheat, Bulgur, Kamut, Oats, Freekeh, and Spelt are also considered whole grains.

LEGUMES

Lentils & Beans are a high source of protein! Try to include them in your diet every day. They are also high in fiber, calcium, and iron.

Don't believe everything you read about gas and beans. There are many things you can do like soaking the beans with a little baking soda and throwing away the soaking liquid.

Another tip, cook a whole peeled potato with the beans. Do not eat the potato and discard before serving. Digestion shouldn't be a problem once you've adapted to the dietary fiber increase. Also, there should be no problem with lentils and chickpeas aka garbanzo beans.

FOR THE CUPBOARD & REFRIGERATOR

- Nutritional Yeast
- Liquid Smoke adds a smokey barbecue flavor to food
- Apple Cider Vinegar
- Cartons of low-sodium Chickpeas
- Cannellini Beans
- Black Beans Grains like quinoa and brown rice
- Sun-dried Tomatoes
- Olives
- Roasted red peppers in the jar
- Cartons of kitchen ready low-salt organic ground tomatoes

- Whole-wheat flour
- Artichokes in water in a jar
- Chickpea Flour

SEASONINGS ARE A VEGAN'S BEST FRIEND!

- Red Pepper flakes
- Sriracha (hot sauce)
- Low-sodium Tamari or Soy Sauce
- Rice Vinegar
- Dried basil
- Dried oregano
- Dried Rosemary
- Dried Thyme
- Ground Chipotle
- Chili Powder
- Cumin
- Onion Powder
- Ground Ginger

FRUIT

Any and all fresh in-season organic fruits. Frozen fruit is also available year-round, and in some cases cheaper than fresh fruit. It also has the same nutritional value.

Fruits like lemons, limes, cranberries, pomegranates, grapefruit, kiwis, pineapple, blueberries, strawberries, and blackcurrants are very low in sugar. Combine them with seeds or a sprinkle of nuts.

**If you have digestive issues, try a cup of warm lemon water when you
wake up in the morning or a half hour before eating**

YOGURT

Any non-dairy yogurt including soy, almond or coconut. I prefer almond. Watch the sweet yogurts for too much sugar. Some yogurts can have over 20 grams of sugar which is not ideal for weight-loss. It also raises your blood sugar too fast. I like to keep the sugar number well below 10 grams.

CREAM CHEESE

You don't have to give up your bagels. Most bagels should be vegan, as the traditional recipe is simply a bread dough that is boiled and baked. Make sure they don't put an egg wash on it to make it shiny. Also ask if they have added any egg, honey or whey to it. A real plain bagel shouldn't have any added ingredients.

There are many vegan cream cheese manufacturers. Check the labels and make sure there isn't too much fat, sodium, and sugar. Remember this is a processed food, so please use sparingly.

ORGANIC VEGETABLE BROTH

I like to use vegetable broth for sautéing instead of added oil. Stock up on organic vegetable broth because you will be using it for many of your soups and stews.

PASTA & NOODLES

Whole-wheat pasta is easy to prepare. Serve with some sautéed chopped tomatoes, sun-dried tomatoes, and basil.

Soba Noodles - cook them in a vegetable broth and top with vegetables.

"ON THE GO" BREAKFAST AND CEREAL

- Natures Path Frozen Waffles (gluten-free, original and flax-plus)
- Barbara's organic breakfast cereal (shredded wheat/multi-grain/whole wheat flakes)
- Instant steel-cut oats (serve with slivered almonds and berries)
- Instant Oatmeal
- Scottish Oats
- Warm farro with organic maple syrup (high-protein)
- Almond yogurt (serve with slivered almonds and fruit for a high-protein breakfast) Warm Quinoa with almond milk, raisins, and chopped fruit

SNACK FOODS

Hummus - Hummus is an excellent high-protein meal. Serve with carrots, cucumber, cherrytomatoes or spread some inside some whole wheat pita bread and top with cucumbers & sprouts.

Whole grain fig bars. Barbara's Raspberry Fig Bars have zero fat.

Whole Wheat Pita Chips -Cut whole wheat pita bread into triangles and put on a cookie sheet.
Roast at 400 until crispy. Serve with salsa or hummus.

Baked sweet potato - Sweet potatoes are loaded with cancer-fighting beta carotene. Wash yoursweet potato, poke some holes in it and bake until tender. Drizzle some maple syrup on top.

Cheesy popcorn - Pop popcorn kernels in an air popper. Transfer popcorn to a large bowl.

Sprinklewith nutritional yeast and mix evenly. Nutritional yeast adds a cheese-like flavor and keeps the crunch of popcorn. Red Star makes a nutritional yeast with a B12 supplement.

Avocado on Whole Wheat Toast - Slice half an avocado and layer on toast. I like to add a littlelemon juice, a touch of salt and sprouts.

Edamame - 6 cups water, 1 pound edamame - Bring water to a boil in large pot. Add soybeansreturn to boil. Cook approximately 10 minutes. Or get the shelled frozen.

Homemade trail mix - Could include raisins, dates, walnuts, almonds and oats. Top with somealmond milk for a quick and easy high protein snack.

Cereal and fruit -Have a bowl of healthy vegan cereal and top it with your favorite berries. Peanut Butter sandwich with sliced banana.

DESSERTS

My favorite dessert is a homemade soft whip banana ice-cream, and it is so simple to prepare: Take two ripe bananas, slice them and put them in the freezer for at least three hours. Then add the frozen banana slices to a food processor with a few cashew nuts, and blend until smooth. Serve with a drizzle of maple syrup and a few chopped walnut pieces.

You can also buy commercial vegan ice cream like:

So Delicious Dairy Free Ice Cream, Purely Decadent Ice Cream and Ben & Jerry's just came out with a vegan ice cream that is delicious.

An ounce of two of 72% dark or bittersweet chocolate *(any chocolate marked over 70% should be non-dairy but check the ingredients)*
Almond pudding cups
Baked fruit with cinnamon and drizzled with maple syrup.
Kid Friendly Vegan Foods
Non-Dairy Yogurt
Peanut Butter & Jelly Sandwiches

Bean and Rice Burritos

Frozen waffles

Whole Wheat Pasta with tomato sauce and ground pine nuts.

Guacamole & Salsa

Baked Sweet Potato Fries

Pancakes

Mac n Cheese with nutritional yeast

Faux chicken fingers with breaded tofu

Hotdogs

(Beware of the ingredients in any processed food especially hot dogs. Check the sodium content and make sure the number representing sodium is lower than the number representing calories. If I had to choose one I think Field Roast Hotdogs taste the best.)

HEALTHIEST PACKAGED FOODS:

The healthiest foods are the foods that come straight out of the garden and are consumed in their natural form or as simply prepared as possible. These foods are fresh fruits, vegetables, starchy vegetables, legumes, and intact whole grains and should be the focus of any healthy diet. Packaged and processed foods are usually loaded with fats, free oils, salt, refined sugars/sweeteners and refined carbohydrates/grains, They are also almost always calorie dense.

However, there are some packaged and processed foods that can be included as part of a healthy diet.

And in fact, keeping some of them around and on hand, can make following a healthy diet, easier.

Organic Frozen Vegetables
Organic Frozen Fruits
Quick Cooking Brown Rice
No Salt added Organic Canned Beans (I like Eden)
No Salt added Organic Kitchen-Ready Tomatoes
Intact Whole Grains (Oatmeal, buckwheat, barley, brown rice, cracked wheat, quinoa, and millet)
Whole Grain Pasta

Organic Dried Fruit

Unsalted Raw Nuts/Seeds & Nut/Seed Butter 10.

Salt-Free Spices/Seasoning & Herbs

BEGIN PLANNING YOUR TRANSITION

This is where you need to seriously think about what is going to work best for you. There are plenty of ways to go vegan you just have to find what's best for you. Here are some common options and some different ideas for ear approach. Find something that appeals to you and tailor it to your needs!

1. VEGETARIAN FOLLOWED BY VEGANISM:

Go vegetarian and then move onto veganism either in one step or by cutting out dairy and eggs one at a time.

MAKING THE TRANSITION:

Remove all meat from your diet, including fish and poultry. Take care not to increase your consumption of eggs and dairy to take the place of meat, focus on including more plant-based protein sources instead.

Pay attention to ingredient lists, avoid products containing gelatin, rennet, and other animal products (excluding dairy and eggs).

If you haven't already, begin incorporating more whole grains, beans, legumes, tofu, nuts, and seeds into your diet.

Once you feel comfortable to move forward you can start phasing out dairy, eggs, and honey. Feel free to do this all at once, one food group at a time, or as slowly as you need to.

2. SLOW TRANSITION FROM OMNIVORE TO VEGAN:

Slowly cut out animal products, starting with the easiest and leaving barrier foods to the end.

Slowly lessen your consumption of animal products while simultaneously increasing the number of plant-based foods in your diet. Continue until you've eliminated all animal products from your diet.

MAKING THE TRANSITION:

Remove any animal products that you won't miss in your diet.

If you haven't already, incorporate more whole grains, beans, legumes, tofu, nuts, and seeds to your diet while simultaneously cutting down on the animal products that you'll miss the least.

You can gradually cut down on all animal products or remove one food/food group at a time.

Remove barrier foods after you feel comfortable with all of the other changes in your diet.

Pay attention to ingredient lists, you may find it easier to begin avoiding the less obvious animal derived ingredients one at a time. You can also choose to overlook them until you've removed all obvious animal products (meat, seafood, dairy products, eggs, etc.) from your diet and you feel comfortable eating mostly plant-based foods.

3. GO FULL-ON VEGAN:

Cut out all animal derived ingredients and incorporate lots of whole grains, beans, legumes, tofu, nuts, and seeds for a healthy vegan diet.

Swap out all of your favourite non-vegan items for vegan alternatives. Many people find that relying on vegan burgers, hot dogs, deli slices, cheeses, etc. can really help ease the transition when cutting out animal products all at once.

MAKING THE TRANSITION:

If you want to dive right in, feel free jump into veganism straight away! You'll want to continue educating yourself so that you're as prepared as possible. For a further crash course in veganism, make sure to learn about:

- How to ensure optimal nutrition on a vegan diet
- How to tell if a product is vegan
- How to build a healthy vegan grocery list
- Budget eating for vegans
- FAQ for new vegans

Some people find relying on vegan alternatives and convenience foods very helpful in easing the transition to veganism. They're often high in protein, fortified with lots of vitamins and minerals, quick and easy to prepare, delicious, and familiar. However, some veggie burgers, veggie dogs, vegan deli slices, etc. are highly processed. Once you begin to feel comfortable with your vegan lifestyle, the use of these products can be lessened. There's nothing wrong with eating the products in moderation, but they shouldn't be used as your main source of vitamins, minerals, and protein for the long-term.

Veganism is much more than a diet, it is a compassionate lifestyle. These guidelines are mostly for transitioning to a vegan diet as that tends to be the most difficult part of becoming vegan. It's also important to learn about vegan alternatives for other products in your life, such as personal care items, clothing, shoes, and other household items.

ALL-OR-NOTHING THINKING & FOOD BARRIERS TO VEGANISM

If you have the desire to become vegan but find yourself struggling with the idea of cravings or giving up a particular food, don't worry, that's completely normal! These are challenges, but they certainly don't have to be barriers. Most vegans stop eating animal products for ethical reasons, not because they don't enjoy the taste of them. It might sound silly but there's lots of cheese-loving vegans out there! (If cheese is your barrier food, read on and then check out our resource: So You Want to Go Vegan but You Love Cheese.)

Far too often people shrug off the idea of veganism for fear of missing a particular food, or they try veganism but end up giving it up in it's entirety for similar reasons. This is often the result of jumping into veganism too quickly with too little preparation. That's why it is so important to take the transition at a pace that works for you so that it's sustainable.

There's a couple of methods that are extremely effective at dealing with these "barrier foods".

LEARN THE PRODUCTION PRACTICES OF YOUR BARRIER FOOD

Learn the ins and outs of how the particular food is produced - this is often enough to turn you off the food for good.

CUT OUT ALL BARRIER FOODS COMPLETELY AND WAIT FOR THE CRAVINGS TO SUBSIDE

Cut out all barrier foods at once. Most people find that cravings for these foods only last a few short weeks and then they subside.

Try slowly introducing vegan alternatives to some of your favourite foods. For some items in particular such as cheese and yogurt you may want to give it a few more weeks before experimenting with substitutions - many people find that the longer it's been since they've had the "real thing", the easier it is for a vegan substitution to satisfy their craving. I found this to be very true for vegan cheese. As a new vegan, non-dairy cheeses didn't do much for me but after a few months of having little bits here and there, the flavour of Daiya really began to grow on me. Now I find it does a great job at satisfying a cheese craving!

You'll also have to find which products you like the most and learn how to prepare them to your liking through a little bit of trial and error.

LEAVE BARRIER FOODS TO THE END OF YOUR TRANSITION

If the idea of becoming vegan appeals to you but you feel like you'll miss a certain food too much to commit 100% to the vegan lifestyle, then start the transition and leave that food until the end. Phase your barrier foods out in a very slow, controlled manner over a few weeks or even months. By this point, you might find that removing the food from your diet is a lot easier than you thought it would be!

If for whatever reason you feel as though you just cannot commit to a 100% vegan diet because of a barrier food, that's okay! Don't let that stop you from minimizing your intake of animal based products to whatever extent you can. Give up all of the animal ingredients and foods that you won't miss, and allow yourself the occasional exception whether it's a food, holiday meal, or favourite restaurant. I advocate following a fully vegan diet and I encourage you to strive towards that as a goal, but it's just silly to abandon veganism in it's entirety because you love bacon or cheese too much. Don't let yourself get caught up in trying to label yourself based on your diet, this is a sort of all-or-nothing thinking that's simply not constructive. If allowing a little flexibility is what will help you sustain a mostly vegan lifestyle then that's exactly what you should do! This also serves to make the vegan lifestyle a lot less daunting and more approachable to others.

HELPFUL HINTS AND REMINDERS

Every little bit counts. Whether you go vegetarian, vegan, or simply cut down your consumption of animal products, you're taking a step in the right direction. Don't let yourself get caught up in trying to label yourself based on your diet.

Don't allow yourself to become overwhelmed. Adopting a vegan lifestyle isn't necessarily difficult, but there is a learning curve. Take your time, expect some mistakes, learn from them, and move on!

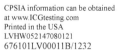
CPSIA information can be obtained
at www.ICGtesting.com
Printed in the USA
LVHW052147080121
676101LV00011B/1232